More Praise for *Forty Bouts in the Wilderness*

With language that is varied and urgent; elegant syntax; and a tone that is both mournful and buoyant, *Forty Bouts in the Wilderness* is a layered story of loss and redemption. Two consecutive miscarriages and a father's recovery from a stroke are at the heart of its braided and recursive narrative.

—Risa Denenberg, author of *Rain/Dweller* and MoonPath Press 2024 Sally Albiso Award judge

Forty Bouts in the Wilderness by Katy E. Ellis embraces grief, disbelief, and acceptance. Reading the first section recalls *Infinite Jest* where the true narrative takes place in footnotes of objective prose. They counterbalance tense tercets in form and tone, fostering a kind of voice-over effect. In the second section, the poet examines her own piety, language, and guilt, attempting to understand how anyone "[comes] to be in this place, in this body, in this life."

—Allen Braden, author of *A Wreath of Down and Drops of Blood*

FORTY BOUTS in the WILDERNESS

FORTY BOUTS
in the
WILDERNESS

Katy E. Ellis

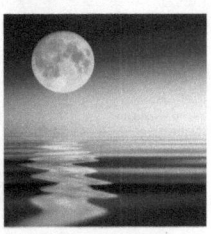

MoonPath Press

Copyright © 2025 Katy E. Ellis
All rights reserved.

No part of this publication may be reproduced, distributed, or transmitted in any form or by any means whatsoever without written permission from the publisher, except in the case of brief excerpts for critical reviews and articles. All inquiries should be addressed to MoonPath Press.

Poetry
ISBN 979-8-9899487-5-8

Cover art: *Quartet by the Pond*,
acrylic painting on wood panel
by Laura C. Thorne
LauratheThorne.com

Author photo: Greg McBrady

Book design by Tonya Namura, using Rawengulk (display)
and Minion Pro (text)

MoonPath Press, an imprint of Concrete Wolf Poetry Series,
is dedicated to publishing the finest poets
living in the U.S. Pacific Northwest.

MoonPath Press
c/o Concrete Wolf
PO Box 2220
Newport, OR 97365-0163

MoonPathPress@gmail.com

http://MoonPathPress.com

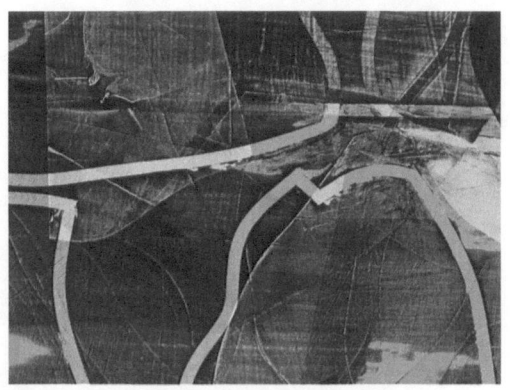

For Greg, the *tender tender*

I am an ignorant pilgrim, crossing a dark valley. And yet for a long time, looking back, I have been unable to shake off the feeling that I have been led—make of that what you will.

—Wendell Berry, *Jayber Crow*

Contents

Forty Bouts in the Wilderness

Pilgrim's Pace

You Were Here	37
The Same Muscle of Unflexed Light	38
The Most Fragile Reappear	41
Dear Istanbul	43
When I Was a New Excommunicant	45
Worthy of Belief	46
Preconceived	48
Signs for Leaving	50
Reading the Wound	52
Years Later I Visit the Night Reservoir	53
Fragments from the New Wilderness	54

[Re]turnings

Gravity	63
I Don't Want to Know the Moon	66
A Place for Uncle Dragon	68
caretaking horses in mexico	70
What Holds the Meadow, the Meadow Also Holds	71
Burning Ground	72
Recurrent	73
Then, a Robin	74
Past Understanding	76
Deciduous	77
Everything for a Reason	78
Bouts Under Sky	79
On Honey Moon	81

When You Grow Up and Read This	82
The Ones Who Walk Again	83
Here	84
Notes	85
Acknowledgments	87
Gratitude	89
About the Author	93

FORTY BOUTS
in the WILDERNESS

bout (noun): 1. A contest between antagonists; a match.
2. A period of time spent in a particular way; a spell.
3. A turning.

{Bouts 1–3}

I answered
to a forgotten name.
My lone voice in the understory.[1]

~

Suddenly—our father
kept alive
by machines.

~

Nurses monitor,
grid and graph our father's
grisly hibernation.

[1] **My lone voice in the understory**: Stories grow one over the other, not as hierarchies but as layers. Understories thrive on loss—the death of a tree stimulates competitive growth in the underbrush. The vegetation of my childhood, for example, stunted by a thick canopy of churchmen, continued to grow past my shunning. Whoever I was or needed or miscarried—started in the dampness of the forest floor, where fern, moss, and fungi swell, where holly and dogwood dance in a ring like boxers in a slow-grow fight for sunlight.

{Bouts 4–6}

~

One sister telephones the lost sister [2]
who climbed unchristened ranges
in search of—

~

A pet name
meaning something between
Little Lamb and *Black Sheep*.

~

Forests of tall monstera
loom at the end
of long, disinfected hallways.

2 **One sister telephones the lost sister**: My sister calls on Valentine's Day, or rather, Valentine's Night. I'm last to arrive, though I speed to the hospital on the hill that overlooks Elliott Bay, skyscrapers tightly huddled nearby. My brothers walk me down the hallway, each resting a hand on my shoulder. When had they last held me in their love? Like two kind police officers, they escort me to our father hooked to machines and a tube draining blood out his skull.

{Bouts 7–9}

~

A person can get lost
not far from holy
water's wash.³

~

The lines of a crayon-drawn map
can take you to the same place
as a store-bought map.

~

Everywhere is somewhere, though
newcomers believed they discovered
the Nowhere of the Northwest.⁴

³ **A person can get lost not far from holy water's wash:** My moon-white christening gown overflowed in Aunt Bonnie's arms. Uncle Bill, my godfather, stood close, while black-robed Pastor three times cupped holy water from the baptismal font and poured it over my soft head. It was never clearly explained to me, the reason my godparents stopped attending our church, but I have an inkling as to why. The pastor was a pompous man who interpreted the scriptures literally. Not ten years later after their leaving I also left the church for good. Some could say we avoided disaster like bobbing boats too near the rocks.

4 **The Nowhere of the Northwest:** Not *nowhere*, but always *now*. And always *here*. Duwamish, Suquamish, Stillaguamish, Muckleshoot. Original inhabitants and stewards of this covered-over tideland at the foot of this hill on which Harborview Hospital stands. A center for trauma for thousands of people from hundreds of miles and years away.

{Bouts 10–12}

~

Almost losing someone
brings to mind
those definitely lost.[5]

~

Did I choose to be lost
—to snake my way
through no man's land?

~

Families claim chairs that unfold into beds,
window seats with views of a distant skybridge to other hospital wings.[6]

5 **Almost losing someone brings to mind those definitely lost:** The last time I'd been in a hospital I delivered a son, born far too soon to live. The blanket the nurse wrapped him in was absurdly big. Like enfolding

a spoon

in a billowing mainsail. *Don't give up*, my father said after this, our second loss. But weren't we already lucky enough? We had a daughter—we wanted more *for her*. Then we wanted more because we lost what we wanted.

6 **views of a distant skybridge**: My family is not the first or only stewards of this ICU waiting room. Others have rearranged chairs into misshapen circles, disarranged the pamphlets. We are not the first to offer one another the open mouths of small bags of chips. Across the room, a family stares at the wall as a young man in their midst softly strums a ukulele. An elderly mother watches her daughter mechanically scroll her phone. A man who can't stay seated for more than three minutes—whose wife's eyes follow him everywhere he paces—gazes and counts the coins in his pocket. We keep forgetting to look out the windows to see how far we are from the ground.

{Bouts 13–15}

~

Over half my life ago
I asked the churchmen how
they knew their God was mine.

~

A single, wild voice
unfurls like the blanket
once used to warm a lost cub.

~

The distance between
sheep in a flock
increases when danger nears.[7]

⁷ **The distance […] when danger nears**: As long as my mom, aunt, sisters, and I never talk about the time I was cast out, we live as forest fairies sipping lilac honey in the light of bluebells.

(Once, I asked my sister where she'd been when I needed her. Where had all the women been?)

Our parents taught us that even if someone tells you they're safe, never eat the wild mushrooms that spring up around the yard or along the forest floor. I remember stomping puffballs in the beauty bark, how the dusty green waft-blasts sent kids running in delightful terror.

(To answer my question, my sister took to bed in tears. She told me later that her husband brought her flowers. Her kids helped make her favorite dinner.)

Yes, there's danger in the understory. And grown men who have cried rivers of wolves for years, who point and shout, *Sheep shredder! Mushroom stomper!*

{Bouts 16–18}

~

I climbed a hundred peaks
heavenward
in search of—

~

A quiet loss.
A compass found.
A missed cross.

~

Which do you prefer:
to lose or be lost,[8]
to fold or unfold?

8 **to lose or be lost**: Imagine crossing west in the early 1800s in a horse-drawn wagon through perilous rockscape and down dizzying, steep trails with your husband and nine children. You are in the first trimester of another reproductive journey. No one has prepared a place for you or your family in the country ahead, though your husband and pastor insist populating this new land fulfills God's plan.

Who drew this map?

When clots of bloody clumps release and seep into your woolen blanket, you feel relief. Your body has given you the gift of loss at the time you needed it most. You praise this body, this omniscient deity. You did not want to carry a tenth child into a new and hostile wilderness. Later you will share this secret gladness in a letter that your dearest friend will hide in the back of a drawer where it is never found.

{Bouts 19–21}

~

Was it punishment for doubt
the Children of Israel were desert-
bound for forty years?

~

I've lived long enough
to know forty years is a long time
to traverse a desert.

~

Depending on the danger,
flocks can be trained
to travel *enfolded*.[9]

⁹ **Depending on the danger, flocks can be trained to travel *enfolded*:** Identifying danger takes as much practice as learning to enfold. As children, we dressed as witches, leopards, or vampires. In blustery darkness, we clustered at each neighborhood door and shouted in unison through our fear of razor blades and poison lacings, demanding sweets with gleeful threats.

When we were in danger of losing our father, I remember my brothers enfolding me again as if nothing had happened in the course of our lives to make them spurn me.

***

I didn't fear losing my first child who turned out to be a healthy daughter, but I did fear losing my life in childbirth. (A common fear, I'm told, in first-time mothers.) So, I taught myself to collect smooth, strong stones. Surrounding me on the day my daughter was born: my husband, and a small flock of chosen women not related to me by blood.

***

When I remember the times I miscarried, I remember nothing of my brothers. They did not embrace me, nor did they speak. Maybe they couldn't imagine a way to enfold a loss their own body could not lose. Or was my loss my punishment—a danger to avoid?

Sensing my distress, I remember my mother and my sisters. They stood in a nearby pasture, bleating mournfully across the strong budding vines of pink-red climbing roses that enveloped the low fieldstone wall I'd built between us.

{Bouts 22–24}

~

Do bears dream[10]
of streams and trails
agleam with snow?

~

Our father speaks
with a bear's voice
from a cave we cannot enter.

~

Bundle the kindling and bones
with silk ribbon.
Lay them at the mouth.

10 **Do bears dream […]?:** I want to hear my father tell his mountain goat dream again. The one where he's hiking the trail we'd once taken together with a gaggle of cousins and brave uncles through thinning alpine forest, along root-stitched valley sides where we walked a narrow high path and told each other to lean against the mountain like it's your mother.

But now is not the time to bother with what he called his *rerun dream*.

Not here in the ICU where he chuffs and growls the wrong order of words to tell me how he met the mountain goat. How he feared his children would fall. How the shaggy beast gathered speed, rushed horns and hooves toward my father pinned to the ledge—

{Bouts 25–27}

~

I named myself
something grey, a middle-born
child among many.[11]

~

Record birth, marriage, death
in the old family Bible.[12]
Leave miscarriage blank.

~

How—
How to carry?
How to carry right?

[11] **middle-born child among many**: I gave myself a secret nickname: *Raincloud*. Grey thing floating overhead at family gatherings. Nimbus on the cusp of crying God's tears into the beer. No longer the bright orange gourd-of-childhood. But *Pumpkin* was decades ago, when my father was the age I am now—standing at his hospital bedside, us children gathered round. He wakes bit by bit. The nurse asks, *Do you know where you are, can you name the president, what is your wife's name and your children?* One by one by one by grey by one.

12 **in the old family Bible**: My father once showed me Blossom, her birthdate and—one day later—her death date written in my grandmother's Bible. Three years later, on Blossom's death date, my father was born. He told me about Robbie, my cousin born with a birth defect, who lived three months and died six months before I was born.

***

Six years after my grandmother died, I quietly miscarried Ribbon, on what would have been my grandmother's eighty-eighth birthday. A little over a year later, I lost a son. I made a small card to mark the day he was born and died. A photo of a blue ceramic tile with the impression of a small boat, passing through, under a riot of stars on a limitless sea. I still calculate his age from the date he should've been born, marking the real years of a child who is only a name.

{Bouts 28–30}

~

Raise your hand if you've prayed
not to beams of sunlight
but to the belly of the moon-chalked night.[13]

~

I wish we would have
named our lost child after a street
not appearing on any map.

~

The same street name
with a different cardinal direction
makes a homonym of place.[14]

13 **to the belly of the moon-chalked night:**   I ask
will I meet my lost son when I die?
    and the moon's answer spills   along the sill
like a barely audible breeze turns picture-book pages
    past the scene of a thumb-sized girl   clutching
the dirty pink ribbon she tied to the dragonfly
    who lifts her free
from a life bound to a slime-mouth toad-in-law—
    the moon's gesso-ready voice brushes me   apart
from the sludge that is my body
    and into the pearl's blue crater
where a child reclines   his palm in mine
    looking up from this night's light
to the moons we don't see

14 **a homonym of place**: My husband and I had planned to name our son after the winding street we traveled down nearly every day to get home. Because of the topography of West Seattle, this street ends at the top of the hill and begins blocks away as a quarter-mile half-turn.

It continues for three-quarters of a mile and over a small bridge across a ravine
                                    and reappears for a two-mile stretch in the up-and-coming industrial part of the city crammed with stadiums and bars—perpendicular to the old Sears & Roebuck building that was conquered by Starbucks, which now houses an Amazon pickup center.

A street that takes me in unwelcome directions—
        his name crosses the city in fits and glimpses.

{Bouts 31–33}

~

Day after day, father bear dormant
in the sanitized fortress where [15]
white shows the dirt my shoes drag in.

~

Let me cobble a crucifix
from coffee stir sticks. Let me dim
this fluorescent light.

~

Remember your gifts
may not always be
welcome.[16]

15 **father bear dormant in the sanitized fortress**: My sister unfurls his fingers, cleans the slough from our father's unused hands. I ask her if she remembers the part in *Big Woods* where Pa feared a tall, burnt stump. How he thought it was a bear because he'd been thinking all the time of bears, afraid he'd meet one.

We are hungry, bleary-eyed children. Where is our father? Where are our uncles? We roam a night cursed by the sound of fluorescent honeybees. A shadow rears up along our trail and I shout into the cave: *Are we brave to fight the shape of our fear? Or foolish to fight a bear?*

16 **Remember your gifts may not always be welcome:** At the time of my baptism, my godparents—Aunt Bonnie and Uncle Bill—were mourning the loss of their infant child, Robbie, who'd died six months before I was born. My own parents had been Robbie's godparents. I imagine my mother and father wanted to return to my aunt and uncle the honor of this role: my helpers and guides to a godly life.

***

The last time I visited my Uncle Bill, he was dying of cancer. I hadn't seen him in years. I tried to lighten the mood by reminding my aunt and uncle that they are my godparents—though we'd all become heathens.

***

They shook their heads disbelieving, said, no, no they didn't remember.

***

Not long after we lost our son, my father snipped a wallet-size image of a baby from a magazine ad and taped it to the windowsill in his overfull office/library/hobby room. Walls crowded with art and quotes, old calendars, and fading pictures of us kids and his blooming array of grandkids. *See this?* He pointed to the glossy, corner-curled baby picture. *That's what I think your little boy would've looked like.*

***

Had he lived, Bonnie's and Bill's son Robbie might've looked like me, standing near my uncle's bedside, dumbly reminding them of who they might have lost.

{Bouts 34–36}

~

Who called me from the dust?[17]
My snowy fleece
once ground in soot.

~

When shouted in canyons
no one's name
returns the same.

~

Swimming in ultrasounds,
the pulse of an altered brain
waves and wanes and wakes.

17 **Who called me from the dust?:**
   Who closed the Valentine and picked up the phone?
   Who said, *I'll be there soon as I can—*
      kissed chocolate from the corners of her child's mouth
      and goodbye-hugged her husband?
   Who forgets terra-cotta pots can crack in winter's freeze?
   Who fears being forgotten just as much as being
      remembered?
   Who (every year) worries she buried
      the tulip bulbs too deep?
   Who crossed the bridge over the still-toxic
      Duwamish River?
   Whose cutout heart got left behind unread?
   Who's unforgiven and who will not forgive?
   Whose God? Who best to ask?
   Who steps into the hospital lobby every time like it's
      the first day of kindergarten?
   Who will surface from the dust bath?

{Bout 37}

~

Asleep.[18]

      Afloat.

Awake.

18 **Asleep**: We wait to see who wakes from father's sleep.
  In this room, hosts of bright fish roam a tank.
I fear the shallows where forget flows deep
  —and I distrust underwater heartbeats.
A county hospital. No shrines. No saints.
  We wait to see who wakes from this unsleep.
Though we don't know if he can hear, we speak
  as if our father hadn't walked the plank.
I fear the shallows where forget flows deep.
  Though I can't name what I've lost, I grieve.
Was I the one who built the ship that sank?
  We wait to see who wakes from this unsleep.
What if my father opens his eyes, sees
  me as stranger among his children's ranks?
I fear the shallows where forget flows deep.
  Brother-sister tides push me out to sea.
A child lost, found, or—? His face a blank.
  I fear I won't survive another sleep
and wade the shadows where forget flows deep.

{Bouts 38–40}

~

No roads. No signs.
It's no wonder
we are lost when—

~

our father reemerges
blinking at the mouth
of a new wilderness and—

~

we leave the ring
to salve our wounds. We wander *Here*
~~unfolded~~ enfolded.

PILGRIM'S PACE

You Were Here

Carve a bowl
from your very bones
and fill it with black earth.

Plant something that resembles you
in eelgrass and alder leaves
and in the cracks of headland rock

where earth's seeds
forever seek and find
rootholds.

Keep elk horn and starfish spoons
alive under your pillow and sleep
near a jar of semiprecious songs.

And when the ink
of your dreams and thoughts
of those dreams

drench a hundred books—
rest. You have etched your breath
in living glass.

The Same Muscle of Unflexed Light

Tell me it was solace—
the three-hour nap on my clean made bed,
my uncanny determination not to wake

though no dreams came.
For night kept not arriving like words
brothers never share.

~

Me, leaving my country
    for the North Star—
goodbye.

Me, slaked of sleep
    willing to wake
shake the marbles in the glass jar
    cat's-eyes to the sky—
come back.

~

Without a confessional it's up to you to decide whether you feel sorry enough to be forgiven. Time can be all it takes. How long in the guilt nest for having sassed your mother? Three hours? Three days? Use your favorite rainbow pencil to write her a note that says *Sorry I was a smart aleck.*

~

Think of the word *requite*.
    Think back.
Think forth.

Is it necessary to repay
    our parents
for what they didn't give?

The word *requite*
    sounds quite nice.

~

Crepuscular: Describing dawn *and* dusk. The same muscle of unflexed light.

~

When the apology notes you write could fill three Plymouth station wagons, you realize that you will always be a *chain sinner*.

~

Think of teeter-totters as scales.
    Does Sister weigh what Brother weighs?
What is each word's mass?

Sin: As much as a lead apron.
    Forgiveness: Equal to dandelion tufts.
Crepuscular: Light as night. Heavy as day.

Reciprocity sounds like a gold rush
    ghost town only tourists visit.

~

In the house nearly empty of everything, you find yourself packing up your mother's top dresser drawer. Here your baby teeth mix with those of your brothers and sisters in a Suisse Mocha International Coffee tin. Here a locket. Mismatched earrings. She saved the notes you girls had written: apologies for acting like a jerk about the dishes or for not cleaning your room after school. You find your letters from Istanbul held together with a rotted rubber band. A photograph of you in front of the Ayasofya. You'd been excommunicated from their church by then. One letter mentions dusk as your favorite time of day—or is it night? For this, you are not sorry.

~
To fly. To breathe underwater.
    To laser-stare a door
through steel or brick. None of these
    powers hold me like my wish
to make my brothers speak.
    Say *goodbye* or come back.
See me in a foreign land, my only armor
    a thick wool sweater-of-many-colors
a smile for the camera
    and seagulls tilt in spins
        past sunset minarets.

The Most Fragile Reappear

In Sultanahmet, the first time we touched,
night slipped like a cat through the window.
Moon-strung courtyard and white laundry ghosts
murmured a halo around her face
as she turned from the night's glow to me.
We kissed as sometimes women do, to bury

a question of love or the need itself to bury.
We'd traveled from Amsterdam, touched
ground once in Beograd's icy station, me
reticent through the train's moving window.
She bellowed and whispered *yes* in the face
of strangeness, of foreign places, of ghosts.

We held hands singing, her body ghosting
mine, and roamed Istanbul with nothing to bury
but the Blue Mosque's wind in our faces
and the starving cats we thought soon touched
by death. I photographed our pensiyon window
not realizing I took a picture of me

standing in a room with no one beside me,
and the photographs would return like ghosts
haunting each framed negative window.
We wanted to see how Muslims bury
their dead, so on our last day we touched
gravestones knowing we now faced

leaving this city which joins the faces
of Europe and Asia. On that day she told me
to love with fists undone, to touch
other people the way stone cloth ghosts
its way around Islamic graves, half-buried
in something deeper than need. Window-

panes steamed with prayer, huge windows
curtained by the eyelids of my new face
opened for a moment, just as before we bury
our dead, the casket yawns and we see. Me,
I unpacked my clothes, washed the ghostly
scent of cats from the cuffs they'd touched.

At home I clean windows and look for me
in the face of the most fragile ghost
that reappears when buried by her missing touch.

Dear Istanbul,

Five months I learned your neighborhoods, heard daily *salat* sail from your minarets, through traffic and alleys, flats and storefronts. I felt you hold and hide me. Now I'm home alone, my family off to church this Easter Sunday, a day to be reminded that emptiness is good, guilt can roll aside and butter the tomb with new light. As you know I was outcast—free to travel countries unknown (and mispronounced)—so my family's church no longer pins me to a weekly service I should not miss. But what I miss is you.

Your countless gulls and crossing boats. Fish with bodies like lungs of an accordion for sale as charms next to Oya & Bora and Cemali cassettes under canvas awnings near the tramway. In Arasta Bazaar, in the shadow of the Blue Mosque, my fingers grazed silk threads of kilims the salesmen unfurled like visions at my feet. Döy Döy Café's *mercimek çorbası*—lentils smooth and warm as blood. I let go the clench of English on my tongue, my language dissolving like the stone Medusa bracing your ancient cistern with a crown of eroded snakes. My skin thickened around the sprig of a new me learning to say please, thank you, *Allahaısmarladık*—I leave you in Allah's care.

Yesterday, my grandparents offered me weak coffee, cookies, and Bible verses. They thought you'd stolen my soul and that your men and mosques coaxed me to stay. Now they believe I've come back to them as the prodigal daughter, who carelessly left the clean sheets and quilts of our family faith hung on the line for the elements to soil. They forgot they found my presence more harrowing than my absence, that my voice no longer harmonizes with the plodding organ pipes that pound Easter hymn-notes like wooden stakes into my heart of doubts.

Once I was a swaddled infant in this room. My mother bathed me in this tub—nearly full now—until I learned to wash myself. I'll think of you, dear Istanbul, as I soak my soul and scrub clean away the dead flesh of the same me who breathed the salt of your Bosphorus air. Until I remember how to be home again. Until I forget how far away I am—

When I Was a New Excommunicant

I used to picture myself deep in the church shrubbery
peering through the colored panes
at my family neat and seated in the pew
behind my grandparents.

I used to want to sing the *kyrie* again
and feel my sister staring at my hair with plans
to curl it special for next Divine Service.
To righteously wilt in Old Testament guilt.

I used to remind myself that I was someone good
at learning by heart every red-lettered word
Jesus spoke in the New Testament. When my pride
burned as a secret I kept from even myself.

I used to imagine them inside reading the note
tied to the rock I wanted to launch through the red glass—
panes reduced to countless slivers sprayed
across the austere altar—my repentance

in the time I used to want their forgiveness.

Worthy of Belief

In Fátima, pilgrims picnicked under oak trees,
bloodied their knees, and bought black-and-white
postcards picturing the three visionary children—
Lúcia, Francisco and Jacinta—in the exact place
Our Lady of the Rosary appeared
as a peace-filled prophetess and a bearer of Light.

I was eighty-six years too late for the light,
for the Miracle of the Sun among sparse trees,
when journalists and doubters began to appear
in the pastureland, under a sky dull white
suddenly purple/scarlet streaked—the place
a knot of moving color. (The core of the children

perhaps made stronger because children
need to be believed in.) I traveled light,
by train, to one of *Lonely Planet*'s holy places.
My unsaid hopes caught like kites in trees,
my daypack filled with baguettes and hard white
Portuguese cheese. I didn't want to appear

only curious—so I made myself appear
more reverent than a tourist, the way a child
notices spectrums between black and white.
Men with useless legs belly-crawled to the lighted
candles encircling a wax Virgin like trees,
and I stood distant and somber, out of place

in this flood of vivid certainty, a dwelling place
for invisible things that will not disappear.
I'd been taught God's presence is common as a tree
—just ask Him for what you want like children
who pose on St. Nick's lap during the season of light
while snow outside buries city streets in white.

But in Fátima I felt intercession's grace in the white
stoked flames of hearts shifting slightly into place
like a time-lapse film of a seed come to light
when spirals burst open and sunflowers appear.
She knows my prayers before I do. Cheering children
untangled kite tails high in the crowns of trees

lining the white-tiled town square. My train appeared
at the wrong time in the right place and like a child
I slept through day's last light, my dreams budding trees.

Preconceived

No Angel Gabriel inflated the room
to announce my womb held a future savior—

but that's what I half expected after years of reliving
the Sunday School story of Mary's fantastic news.

In tissue-paper Bible pages and TV specials I felt
incarnation saturate the atmosphere with a pregnancy

of light to redeem women whose wombs might
someday expand with a kaleidoscope of cells.

Stories of women precisely knowing
the moment of conception occurred when stirring

beef barley soup, when walking to work past city hall
or upon waking after a dream of robins.

That spring I lay atop a stone cliff
on the Portuguese coast near succulents bearing

ludicrous hot-pink blooms in the crags. There
I beseeched the Atlantic and God, of course, in prayer:

*Please, give me a child now or at least
let me know if it will never happen.* I always thought

there'd be more than a woman opening
eggs between her legs—the tug and drain of a million

twinkles in a man's eye scattering like buckshot.
Something more like the pour of moon

against a woman's cheekbone or a man's forearm.
Something more than ovulation, disorganized orgasm.

I took a feverish while to know a speck, a bean, a prawn
began basket-weaving three-hundred translucent

bones of hope near memory of basalt against my spine
where no wings or voices had ever touched me.

Signs for Leaving
Ericeira, Portugal

The stone spoon
    you carry in your pocket
speaks—its concave a small mouth
    a thumb rest. *Why*

are you here? When sun opens
the souvenir shops again—
it's the end of the deafening
season of wind. *You are here*

because you don't know where else
to be. Hold the spoon high
by its amber-veined neck—
to stir the air like shadow flocks.

    Westward, two groups of birds
    form separate lasso circles.

    They do not make
    a figure eight.

You know there's nothing here
to feed your broken houses
where roots and rising tides
muscle through foundations.

Nothing to leave
on the café table

but a trio of coins
in a currency worth

    two waterless eyes

    a spatter of scales

    a handful of rib

    bones too thin to whittle

Reading the Wound

Gutting avocado when the knife
slips through a lifeline. The open hand
a sudden live-stream map
charting the course of a red river.

Spirit, travel, marriage, luck:
one knife dragged across these lines
and life in the palm
of what is meant to be
                        disappears.

But if it was that simple
wouldn't we all choose
scars and grafted skin
to cover the bad luck line

extend the deep wrinkle of travel and marriage
add or erase
the spirits of children
we're to bear?

Some endings will happen this way—
    the fruit's round pit like a lazy pinball
    bumps the chair leg, stops half-
    way across the kitchen's linoleum field

Years Later I Visit the Night Reservoir

This man-made lake takes
                          my breath

over the surface   to the other side
where a train hauls fallen stars and scrap metal.

They say an eight-hundred-year-old cedar
takes eight hundred years to decompose.

Do they say a nineteen-year-old girl who leaves home
takes nineteen years to return as someone recomposed?

I've come back. And I (standing
on what feels like a nature-made shore)

recall my old excommunication
how the first syllable made an X

through the church-made faith
I questioned half my life ago.

Now I know this water fills or empties as needed
like breath or blood   a dream or a stone.

I know that train   now tracing
the opposite shore of what looks like a real lake

pulls through me—
like a meteor's tail thread

of living light.   Again
I am.

Fragments from the New Wilderness

In one of many follow-up appointments, we learned the three layers between brain and skull: *dura* (tough) *mater*, *arachnoid* (spiderlike) *mater*, and *pia* (tender) *mater*. These layers act as a strong pouch, the doctor told us, enveloping the brain to keep the treasure safe. After his aneurysm and massive stroke, my father told anyone who would listen, *Did you know I keep my brain in a pouch?*

~

Mater: "mother" (Latin).

~

At Ye Olde Curiosity Shop on the Seattle waterfront, my husband and I let our five-year-old daughter choose a handful of polished stones from a rustic wooden cart. She chooses three rose quartz, one crackly amethyst, and a rough, frosty green stone (the name of which we never learned). She places the stones in a tiny, complimentary velvet sack, pulls the drawstring tight, and does not look at her precious take until we are safely home.

~

Dura mater: "tough mother." Outermost, protective membrane layer that envelops the brain and spinal cord.

~

When my friend's young son overheard her telling someone that I'd *lost the baby*, he couldn't fathom how in the world I could lose a baby. *Where did she look?* He wanted to make sure I'd searched the whole house.

~

The neurologist warned us of *perseveration*: the involuntarily repetition of a thought, phrase, or behavior despite the absence of the original, triggering experience or thought (often to an extreme degree). For instance, the battles at Fort Ticonderoga and repetition of the word Ticonderoga after handing my father a Ticonderoga #2 pencil. Or hours of concern for the demise of receipts left fluttering next to fuel nozzles at gas pumps.

~

Did you know I keep my brain in a pouch?

~

In our confusion and fear we searched for the nearest container to hold this sudden loss of vein and helix, a festoon of cells only vaguely human-shaped. I point above our coats in the open hall closet across from the bathroom. My husband empties the box marked *Ribbon*.

~

Arachnoid mater: "spiderlike mother" (Latin). Named for the fine, spiderweb-like appearance of the delicate fibers which attach to the pia mater and help circulate cerebrospinal fluid between arachnoid and pia mater, and flow freely through the nervous system.

~

Out tumbled spools of magenta satin ribbon, the polka-dotted ribbon from our daughter's first birthday, long strands of thin green ribbon, and a jumble of other colored and textured ribbons that I can never stop myself snipping from racks at the card shop or fabric stores. At family parties I stealthily snag a yard here or there from the cast-off piles of wrapping paper.

~

They removed and cryogenically preserved a piece of my father's skull until the swelling in his brain subsided. The right side of his head bore an obvious indentation outlined by a horseshoe-shaped incision held together with staples. He lightly circled and circled the suture with his index finger as if deciphering a brailled clue as to how he came to be in this place, in this body, in this life.

~

Of the five chosen stones in our daughter's new collection, rose quartz is her favorite. She names her pet fish—a White Cloud Mountain minnow—after the stone. Overfed Rose Quartz swims in a small tank with faux sea plants. A hardy species, White Cloud Mountain minnows are virtually extinct in their native habitat, but can survive and even flourish in cold, unfiltered fish tanks on a child's dresser for years on end.

~

When can I go back to my real home? My father whispered to me a week after his hospital discharge, when I'd stopped by to visit. *You're home now*, I said. He timidly studied the front room of the house he'd lived in for forty-eight years, nodding at the striped couch, the painted bluebirds on the ceramic lamp, the woodstove. *Looks like it but doesn't feel like it.* When I asked him what it felt like, he said, *Not home.*

~

Rose quartz is often called the Love Stone. They say it is the stone for every type of love: self-love, family, platonic, romantic, and unconditional. A rose quartz in your pocket can not only bring inner warmth, it lowers stress and soothes the air around you.

~

Pia mater: "tender mother" (Latin). The delicate innermost membrane enveloping the brain and spinal cord, the pia mater is a thin fibrous tissue that is permeable to water and small solutes. The pia mater allows blood vessels to pass through and nourish the brain.

~

Did you feed Rose Quartz today?

~

My sister kept a three-ring binder with our father's hospital discharge papers, medication information, instructions for his various cognitive and physical rehab exercises. He'd ask, *Does it say in there what happened to me? When will they announce what happened?* Of course, we explained it many times—the aneurysm, the ambulance to Harborview Hospital, the brain bleed, and the stroke. In our retelling we add more detail as if convincing him, as if the story of what happened to our father is a new path we tamp on the surface of our own brains.

~

A schoolmate tells our daughter that an amethyst under your pillow gives happy dreams. She places the amethyst under her pillow. She adds her three pink stones so that happy amethyst dreams will be accompanied by rose quartz love.

~

At times it wasn't a dream but an automatic image whenever I closed my eyes:

    I'm on the side of a treeless mountain

        looking into a waterway between islands.

    When I stretch out my arms and open my hands

ribbons of all colors and textures unspool

    endlessly

        from the center of my palms.

A steady wind pulls iridescent blue-indigo ribbon

    away from me and into the currents of the sky—

~

When can I go back to my real home?

~

We tried again after the time of Ribbon. Past the halfway point, we thought we were in the clear: Heartbeat. Sex revealed in ultrasound. *Size of an ear of corn.* Somersaults.

Prenatal yoga classes. Daycare waitlist. Name. We thought this time we were in the clear.

~

Chorion: "skin" (Greek). The outer layer surrounding the embryo of reptiles, birds, and mammals and which forms the placenta.

Amnion: "bowl to catch the blood" (Greek). A thin layer forming a closed sac about the embryo or fetus of a reptile, bird, or mammal and containing a watery fluid.

~

They say ancient Egyptians used the amethyst to guard against guilty and fearful feelings.

~

Chorioamnionitis: an intra-amniotic infection of the chorion and amnion; loss likely caused by not being a good daughter, mother, sister, or wife or by greed (e.g., wanting more than one healthy child) or by not being worthy, healthy, or clean enough; a rightful punishment for leaving the church as a young woman; bad luck; an infection of layers.

~

Amethyst can also be worn as protection from self-deception.

~

~~The most intricate strings of magenta and moss green and marigold unspool from my hands, lift in the wind, sail over the watery trails between island mounds and I can't tell if I'm holding on to an end, if there is no end, or if these ribbons connect me to that place.~~

~

This one's too special for us to see, my daughter says of the unnamed green stone. She tucks it safe in its dark little pouch.

[RE]TURNINGS

Gravity

One
When Valeri Polyakov returned
after four hundred thirty eight days in space
his heart began again the work
of moving blood through veins
because on Earth there's up
and down.

After so much time in space
would I then believe
that heaven sinks below
and hell burns blue?

Two
On Earth weight comes and goes.

As I lie at the foot of a hot springs
high tide fills the lower rock pools
in waves. I weigh
just bone and skin,
heart and lungs,
the picnic lunch and every memory
of someone inside my body.

Then slowly I weigh nothing:
salt water,
    glass ball,
        space.

Three
To demonstrate the moon's pull
on oceans, on wombs
I tilt the spilt
tea in my saucer
around, around and
consider the great, fixed gulf we cannot stretch
between the beggar's cool water
and the rich man's blistered tongue.

Four
I confuse the facts
by the gravity I place upon them:

    A tide chart hangs by my door.

    At certain times of day china shards,
    blue glass, starfish, sludge and barnacles
    appear at Dolphin Point.

    At certain times of day
    Dolphin Point does not exist.

    If I'm good
           I'll go Up—
    Down
           if I'm bad.

    My belly swells in anticipation.

    I cry easily.

Five
When he entered his old atmosphere,
gravity yanked Valerie Polyakov
through Earth's blue shroud
and sidewalk clouds
and further down
the skyscraped skin
that holds our breath
                      until he pierced
another spacious ocean
brimmed in salt
and stars.

I Don't Want to Know the Moon

From the Space Needle
ten-cents-a-minute viewer
I don't see a face or a rabbit
in the moon's sea.
No man or woman
covered in lunar bits and star nits.
There's a belly button maybe
stretch—birth—or beauty marks.
Nothing spelled out except C is a cup.
But is it pouring out light
or filling up?

I don't see golden anything
but plums the first time
I wrap my naked self in sheets,
barefoot through the orchard
to cull low branches
for moonlight-sweetened full fruit.
Blue wine beneath moths
in compulsive love with landing
and dying on light bulbs.

What is all this about tektites
and hard candies pelted
from orbital distances?
Or grazing occultation
—a body's edge touched and untouched?
Don't tell me about earthshine—
old moon in the new moon's arms—
cradles illuminated.

The last thing I need to know is
the dark side exists—every crater
a named mouth: Apollo, Tsander,

Korolev, Mendeleev.
The moon does not bear children,
or secretly howl behind itself.

It's enough for me to know
my moon was first named
Young Birds Are Full-Fledged,
Sturgeon, Green Corn
and Berries Ripen
Even in the Night
Moon.

A Place for Uncle Dragon

I stitched these berries for you
out of Easter grass and broken eggshells—
     taste their rose salt.

Your front porch steps
now lead to the paper cave I folded for you
damp with lake water where we swam
at the company picnic.

If you guess which fist holds
the watermelon seed
     you may step up one.

This time
the right hand is empty

and the left hand opens
a door I draped in sea lettuce, heavy
with the fishy smell of low tide.

Inside, the house is wide and quiet as fire's light.

Your hooves ache.
You've walked the land so long
your vestigial wing bones throb.

I rigged the plumbing here
to make mountain ranges overflow your tub.
Soak now, Uncle, in a bath of Cascade and Sawtooth.
Mesabi Iron will rinse you clean.

When the kindling dwindles our last hymn to ashes,
I'll make a place for you to sleep:
    a nest of guitar strums
    a whorl of milkweed silk
    a cigarette from thin air

caretaking horses in mexico

it's a land of many bridges but there's no water to cross
    dust flails on gold-flecked beaches   empty pails
dogs on three legs and parched

we want to remember names on crosses
    invisible rapids   silent in this months-long ebb
of pieced-together mirage towns   scrap metal
    and burlap bags   where the forgetting season flows

always thirsty to know our earthly coordinates
    we click reverent photographs of *trópico de cáncer*—
latitude proof we touched that famous notch
    on one of our globe's imaginary belts   but why

care about landmarks?   our place is among the horses
    helping shovel manure   refill troughs
and launch crackers of hay into the corrals

our days: voluminous sun   our nights: whole moons

when we return to the office people will ask us
    to pinpoint the ranch on a map of the baja peninsula
we will shrug and say

it was near a mountain that changed names
    depending on the direction we came from
        and a dry riverbed
            we never followed
to the spring

What Holds the Meadow, the Meadow Also Holds

They waded chest high when the foreteller ducks began
diving into the loose weave of underwater rhizomes.

No one knew scientifically how essential the diatoms.

No one referred to the pollen as filamentous
though it gave light. They listened as eelgrass

spoke in waves—heard rot give birth to flesh.

Ninety years later, us kids learn tadpoles once choked
a small creek on this land now crowned with a strip mall.

Horses grazed tall fescue under this black-tar parking lot

chewing in tune to the hum of moss-caked boulders.
We change dollars for tokens to conquer

ghosts that threaten our yellow video-globe lives.

Burning Ground

We couldn't see blood hemorrhaging across the grasslands
of our father's right brain hemisphere like a fiery
saw blade on the horizon, separating

land/smoke
father we know/don't know.

No time for us to dig a moat around the family history
built on a one-way train ticket from Duluth to Seattle
and the oldest Luedtke girl cashiering at Schrader Drugs.

No choice what's saved/what's lost
of his memory store.

He recalled a love of cold milk but couldn't name the thing
that tells time that you wear on your wrist. Lost
the steps for tying shoes, yet in capital letters

he wrote and correctly spelled
the name of each grandchild.

We had to trust the small fires we lit
when our father knew us as his children.
Pray our flames burned ground enough to keep

the father who remains/
the father we mourn.

Recurrent

When fields and forests held
more territory than the homes
and new apartment complexes
of our suburban neighborhood
we kids used to maze paths
through the timothy, fescue
and orchardgrass that surrounded
a broken farmhouse on a low hill
near our elementary school. I remember
flattening a circle in the grass like a nest
to curl my body inside. Only
the sun or the pale daymoon could see me.
This is where I lie
once again next to my lost son
who nurses ghost milk for hours
from my mourn-full breasts
until I wake.

Then, a Robin

In our raw loss, new absence
burrowed quickly to rearrange the loam.

We three had come from the beach—
my husband, our girl, and me
—with prayers on our lips
and a handful of shells touched
by candle wax

when a robin twitched the ivy wall
and caught our daughter's eye.

Only the day before
she'd reluctantly confessed a wish
to find a bird with a broken wing
to care for in a little box
in her bedroom.

So we brought the robin home instead
of the newborn boy we'd been expecting

to swaddle into our lives. Tiny water dish,
a single raspberry, a fleecy blanket nest.
By morning her robin had sprung from the box
chirping *Alarm!* to the birds on the eaves
outside the open bedroom window.

Before we left him in the understory
of the hillside forest behind our house

she held the robin—
not like a handful of wild blackberries
not like cupped ocean water

skeleton shrimp darting the palms
—she held him like a labored love accomplished

a care she could now
let the trees take.

Past Understanding

If our masks defend us from both
seasons of fire and virus,
then we will walk to the trees again

inhale the atmospheric grit—grey
and ghostly as a forest gone to ash.
We'll welcome fog as breathable water.

If our mother's eye shines in, seeking
our source of soreness and red rasp
we'll concede her declaration of unwellness.

If the stomach is a rib-encircled pond
that holds sorrow like a dark bowl
then we will *Drink*

a warm mug of water with or without
a squeeze of lemon each morning first thing—
to soothe our undigested wishes.

We will crawl to our heart's cul-de-sac,
turn nose to tail like a dog circles
before lying down to sleep.

Deciduous

A child might lose the first one in Earth Science
where they spend twenty minutes a week
observing nature shows on TV.

It may or may not be a surprise to finally hold
the chalky white seed touched with blood
between unsanitized fingers.

The deciduous teeth don't *fall* out like people say they do.
They don't break loose suddenly
and twirl to the ground like sycamore propellers.

They cling by porcelain threadroot until
                    something clicks—
a cup in the gums fills with newborn white.

Many mothers can't stomach the losing.
After all, the deciduous were partly her creation
plucked now, twisted out, wiggled

free from that old womb place,
that pouch outgrown
several gasping springs ago

when it was and was not a surprise to wince
at the clamped demand
of tooth buds blooming new. All children lose

their mouthful of charms. Some swap teeth at night
for dulled silver dimes, a Matchbox car
or a strand of secondhand pearls.

Everything for a Reason

In church I learned that luck is a sin
when confused with blessings.
Better to hang a silver Jesus-
fish on my neck chain
than to hammer horseshoes
above my door.

Pray. (And worry not—God
orchestrates all happenstance.)

Prayer is an act of worship, a give
and take between the lips
or between the sacred covers
of childhood diaries: *Please, God,
forgive me asking for things I don't deserve.*

My oldest brother taught me
how to watch a baseball game
rooting for a team that almost never won.
After the first time I witnessed
my first bases-loaded homer
I prayed like a secret devil
making deals for grand slams.

Who in their life hasn't ached
for a miracle win?

Eyes closed, my worship bore
a decent amount of human hope
always sprinkled with *Thy will be done*
to guard against visions of heavenly coins
twinkle-flipping to Earth, landing
wrong side-up on my head.

Bouts Under Sky

An open dish of nighttime
kibble set out
beneath the eaves.

~

God arrives in adolescent hearts
bearing a name
young girls do not choose.

~

Whose daughter unprays—
turns her palm's
old blisters to green boughs?

~

Remember the litter of kittens
all you kids wanted to rescue
—especially the runt.

~

It takes courage to know
returning is the blanket
ache and cure.

~

Pull wide the corners of brother/sister fold.
Lie down—become
a love-held bundle of one's own.

~

When Father's eyes next open
he sees me, asks
do you still climb trees—

~

*—I gave you a boost
when you couldn't reach
the first rung in a ladder of branches.*

~

My human father is the *other
god* I worshipped
before the first Thou Shalt Not.

~

When we hold hands
lifelines churn
in temporary confluence.

~

One daughter teaches her daughter
to call God out in the forest, receive
pieces of sky and falling sun.

~

The map I drew leads home
where abandoned kittens
thrive door-to-door in starlight.

On Honey Moon

He bicycles into a bee—
gets stung
with surprise

like the small electrostatic
shock of kissing someone
who often drags her feet.

It stuns me—his calm
stop to scoop grey clay
onto his swelling lip

as if anyone could
grasp earth's power
to draw out venom.

Five married years later
I'll gape again
at his instinct to gather

our undone mud selves
and mound our missing
pieces into poultice.

He peddles on with me
down graveled crater lanes
pointing out marsh orchids

a swayback horse
the ruins of stone church
—both of us certain

there'll be more honey
more hive
less sting.

When You Grow Up and Read This

I will have given you my best necklaces,
the orange rhinestone choker
with matching earrings, and all the gifts
of well-thought-out love
your father gave me.

Among those stones and clasps
there will be an apology
there will be hope that you've forgotten
the sister-wish of ribbons
and the little brother
who never came home.

Hope that all along you felt
you were enough for us and filled
our house like Angel Gabriel's gown of light
pushing out the windowpanes.

When you read this, touch your throat
where air sweeps alive
your beautiful trachea
your sailcloth lungs.
Feel your breath lift green glass beads
faceted amethyst
each ring of silver on the long chain
where I hang a lighthouse, a Tahitian pearl
or a compass—each morning
choosing a talisman more than
lucky enough.

The Ones Who Walk Again

A Duwamish man told the story
to my daughter at a school assembly.
He drummed in a world
of children who walk into the water
and who return as Salmon
for the villagers to eat.

Now she worries beyond reason
for the Salmon boys and Salmon girls—
the ones who will not walk again
should the drying bones of our last night's dinner
not be returned to sea.

Always the ocean down our street
keeps up its chop and spit and rush
and I pay bills, sack lunches, wash clothes
in cycles spinning my hand-me-down myths
—the ones I will not give her.

She plucks each bone of a heart-held story
from the dish in her hands
and feeds them to the waves that slosh
against her legs like underpinnings
of a miles-long pier.

Here

      They call it *earthing*—
to pad along shoeless, prying fear
from between curled toes.

      My bare feet
pulse tandem to shorelines.
      My blood

follows me
from Minnesota roots
to the puddle chest:

rain waxes   the moon
evaporates pondwater.
      My own bones

make the moss-limb
house of my new backyard.
      I'm no more scolded

for running naked of shoes
for living as if there were no stingers,
glass shards, dog shit, pine pitch.

      Now feel: egg-print heel
pressed to sand
or river mud, mark both

sole and soul.
      I *earth*
into place.

Notes

As a counter note to the first footnote **my lone voice in the understory** in the title poem *Forty Bouts in the Wilderness*, which emphasizes competitive growth in the forest, there is an abundance of research and writing, particularly in Suzanne Simard's *Finding the Mother Tree* (Alfred A. Knopf, 2021), pointing to the communicative, cooperative, and supportive nature of forest ecosystems from soil to understory to canopy.

"Fragments from the New Wilderness" uses definitions found through various internet searches. These definitions have been edited and formatted to suit the needs of the poem and should not be used for diagnosis. Maybe use WebMD for that?

The second to last line from "You Were Here" has stuck with me for many years and was taken from a section of Susanne Antonetta's book *A Mind Apart: Travels in a Neurodiverse World* (Penguin, 2007): *Marcus Aurelius writes that the sole life we can lose is the one that we live at this moment, and we can have no other life than that which we lose: so the longest life, and the shortest, amount to the same. Live to be a hundred, die at birth: just a few heartbeats etch you in the glass of the living.*

The form of "The Same Muscle of Unflexed Light" mimics the poem "On Earth We Are Briefly Gorgeous" in Ocean Vuong's book *Night Sky with Exit Wounds* (Copper Canyon, 2016).

"A Place for Uncle Dragon" is dedicated to the memory of my Uncle Bill, my mom's brother, who was born April, 5, 1943, and died at home from cancer on July, 29, 2013.

Acknowledgments

The author wishes to acknowledge and thank the following publications where some of the poems in this collection previously appeared, some in earlier versions.

Alehouse: Poetry on Tap: "Signs for Leaving"

American Journal of Poetry: "The Same Muscle of Unflexed Light"

CALYX: A Journal of Art and Literature by Women: "The Most Fragile Reappear"

Gravity (chapbook, Yellow Flag Press): "Gravity"

I Sing the Salmon Home: Poems from Washington State (anthology, Empty Bowl Press): "The Ones Who Walk Again"

MER (Mom Egg Review): "Deciduous"

Pontoon: "Then, a Robin"

Seattle Review of Books: "Here"(online as part of featured poet of the month)

SWWIM Every Day: "Burning Ground"

Urban Animal Expeditions (chapbook, dancing girl press): "I Don't Want to Know the Moon"

The poem "Deciduous" received Honorable Mention for Carlow University's Patricia Dobler Poetry Award.

The poem "Gravity" was nominated for a Pushcart Prize.

Gratitude

Much of this book was written while I lived in a little rented duplex with my husband, Greg, and our young daughter, Qwynn, in a sea-level neighborhood near Alki Beach in West Seattle. That area is the ancestral home of the Duwamish Tribe who to this day have not received federal recognition of tribal sovereignty that predates the history of the United States (read more here: www.DuwamishTribe.com). I'm grateful for that time in which I walked (and walked and walked) along the water, following the contours of Alki Point and looking out at Puget Sound. That place healed and held me.

Thank-you to my writing group—who read many early drafts of these poems: Chris Balk, Michele Bombardier, Suzanne Edison, Susan Landgraf, Susan Rich, and Cindy Veach. Always, always thank you to Ann Teplick. My deep appreciation to Susan Landgraf for reading this manuscript with an eagle eye to provide insightful edits and revisions. To MoonPath Press Editor Lana Ayers for helping me push through my "late bloomer" doubts.

Special thank you to Heather Simeney MacLeod who taught me to separate writing poems and submitting poems. To not let rejections—no matter how many!—hold me back from writing more and submitting more. Thank you for your incredible friendship, love, and unwavering support and encouragement of my writing.

I'm grateful to Susan Tower and Laura Thorne (early readers of the poem "Forty Bouts in the Wilderness") for your eternal sisterhood and friendship, for reading and supporting my work in ways you don't even know. Thank you, Laura, for enthusiastically allowing me to use your art for my book cover(s). I will forever be buoyed and intrigued by your visual art; how you see and paint this world; how you have always been willing to dedicate your living space to your living art.

To the Luedtkes: Aunt Bonnie and Uncle Bill, my cousins Bill, Jeff, Mike, Jon, and Liz. Thank you, Aunt Bonnie, for your willingness to talk about Robbie's short life and for letting me share some of your story in this book. Special thanks to Sarah Luedtke for unfailingly saying what needs saying (and what needs to be laughed at) and for reaching out with encouragement, generosity, and kindness.

I'm grateful to the doctors, nurses, and other specialists at Harborview Medical Center for their care and expertise. What a gift to have so many years with my dad after his stroke, which also gave me the chance to connect in new ways with my sisters and brothers as we worked together (and still do) to care for our parents.

Deep thanks to my friends and family who took care of me, Qwynn, and Greg when we needed help, I cannot thank you enough. Special thanks to Janine Lange for understanding and counselling me when I needed it most.

To my Bellingham Crew: Rob Whitner, Janelle Gavin, Kathryn Place (née Kowalski), Bobbi Ewing, Mike Falcone, Rebecca Brown, Dave Lister, Kami Westoff, Bruce Beasley, Carol Guess, and Suzanne Paola. Meeting and learning from each of you renewed my love and need to write. Thank you for your continued friendship, encouragement, hospitality, and wild humor.

Mountains of thanks to the communities and friends who continually attend readings and support my poetry in the world especially Micha West—my Alki "loop" walking partner, Cecyl and Rick Fabano, Jeani George

(Jacob, Rowan, and Adrie too), Alan Greenbaum, Cause Haun, Stephanie Koura, Janine and Jon Lange, Mary Marin, Linda Martinez, John Overton, my Public Health—Seattle & King County friends and teammates, all the incredible WordsWest attendees who keep coming back (and to Susan Rich and Harold Taw, co-curators of that magical literary series), and to the poetry writers and readers of Vashon Island.

And, as always, thank you to Greg and Qwynn for letting me be my whole self with you no matter where we roam. It amazes me that you both will read or listen to my poems and give your feedback at the drop of a hat. Thank you for sharing your lives with me—an experience that continually improves the quality of my life every day.

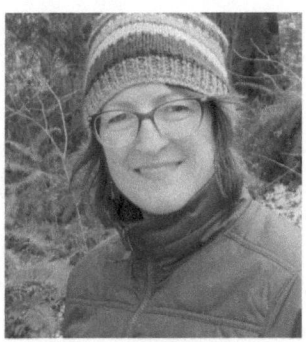

About the Author

Katy E. Ellis is the author of the novel-length prose poem *Home Water, Home Land* (Tolsun Books) and three chapbooks, including *Night Watch*, winner of Floating Bridge Press's 2017 John Pierce Chapbook Competition, *Urban Animal Expeditions* (Dancing Girl Press), and *Gravity* (Yellow Flag Press).

Her poetry appears in a number of print and online literary journals and anthologies including *I Sing the Salmon Home: Poems from Washington State*, *Till the Tide: An Anthology of Mermaid Poetry*, *Mom Egg Review* (*MER*), *SWWIM Every Day*, *Pithead Chapel*, *The American Journal of Poetry*, *Literary Mama*, *MAYDAY Magazine*, *CALYX: A Journal of Art & Literature by Women*, *Borderlands: Texas Poetry Review*, and the Canadian journals *PRISM International*, *Grain*, and *Fiddlehead*. Her fiction has appeared in *Burnside Review* and won Third Place in the *Glimmer Train* super-short fiction contest. She has twice been nominated for a Pushcart Prize.

She received a Bachelor of Arts degree studying creative writing at the University of Victoria's Fine Arts Program in Victoria, British Columbia, Canada, and a Master's Degree in English with a creative writing emphasis at Western Washington University, in Bellingham, Washington.

For five years Katy co-curated WordsWest Literary Series, a monthly literary event in West Seattle. She has been awarded grants from the Elizabeth George Foundation, Seattle's Office of Arts & Culture and Artist Trust/Centrum. Learn more at www.KatyEEllis.com

www.ingramcontent.com/pod-product-compliance
Lightning Source LLC
LaVergne TN
LVHW041617070526
838199LV00052B/3175